Worthy

WORTHY:

OVERCOMING TRAUMA, HEALING, AND FINDING GRATITUDE AND SACRED MEDICINES

HEALINGLIVMAMA LOVE

This book is dedicated to anyone who has ever questioned their worth. You are worthy. To anyone who has ever felt unwell, you are capable of healing.

I was an exceptionally awkward, self-conscious, sensitive child. A middle child to an exceptionally bright, ambitious, and academic father and a mentally ill stay-at-home mother who was overburdened by the task of caring for three children, I found solace and escape through books. They were my original portal to another reality, and I soaked up as much as I could, burying myself ceaselessly in reading as much as I could manage.

While I felt sympathetic toward my mother's plight, I was also determined not to be like her and used to proclaim as a child that I would one day earn a Ph.D., following in my father's footsteps. I am now a 40-year-old single mother, A.B.D. (All But Dissertation), in the middle of writing my dissertation, and still mourning my father's death, may his spirit rest in peace. My father was an astoundingly accomplished, prolific academic, entrepreneur, and visionary in the field of AI and machine translation. Now that he is gone, I find myself questioning whether I really want this Ph.D. and even more so, whether I can envision myself staying in academia professionally. My father, who had reached the pinnacle of success in academia, is now deceased, at only 66 years old after a protracted battle with cancer; do I really want to follow in a similar trajectory?

Mostly, I find myself wondering how to balance parenting, work, and wellness, and what that will look like given my current unmoored state and the liminal state of the world.

I am sure that, just as everyone has contemplated suicide, everyone has, or has had, those moments of being convinced that they are not worthy. The imposter syndrome, but more than that, a sense of deep unworthiness. As a child and even through my 20's and early 30's, I found myself continually questioning whether I was worthy. Years of therapy and exposure to the wellness community have taught me that much of this stems from my childhood. Well, *duh*. In my early childhood years, my mother almost exclusively dressed me in hand-me-downs from my brother, which led me in second grade to start wearing only dresses. I still vividly recall my entire class standing up to applaud for me the first time I walked into the classroom wearing jeans, after my extended, years-long phase of only wearing dresses. Though I always had thought of myself as inherently shy, I've gained tremendous perspective from being a parent that this was also clearly related to my being neglected and not well-socialized as a young child. My dad was busy with his professional and personal pursuits and absent much of the time, and my mom did not work outside of caring for her children. My parents had always been exceptionally miserly, and we had always thought of ourselves as poor. My siblings and I also only rarely ever had babysitters, and we were exceptionally shy from such an insular and impoverished upbringing. And so of course the stigma, shame, and trauma of those formative childhood years indelibly left their marks on me.

Add to our neglect and my general unkempt state an auto-immune condition that left my skin constantly flaring up and my allergies triggered, and you can understand why it took me literally decades to overcome my awkwardness and self-consciousness. I thought of myself as intrinsically inferior, with bad genes (not only my skin and allergies but also unruly, thick curly hair and a proportionally large nose) and a legacy of perceived poverty due to my parents' extreme, even irrational frugality, that I've long since struggled to shake off. Eczema plagued me throughout my childhood; at least one finger was perpetually so inflamed that it would crack open and bleed. I frequently tried to cover up my flare-ups with Band-Aids, and my condition caused me so much self-consciousness and shame that I got into the habit of hiding my hands in embarrassment much of the time. I would also get rashes behind my knees in the summer, aggravated by the heat and humidity, but this was nothing compared to the persistent cracked skin on my hands that caused me endless embarrassment and shame. These unsightly, itchy flare-ups persisted through the years despite countless visits to the pediatrician and dermatologists, and despite the regular use of various cortisone ointments and creams. My mom was dutiful in taking me to the doctor, but, stuck in her Western paradigm, she had never considered addressing possible causes or trying anything outside of a conventional approach to help me.

From what I remember, though I could have simply been paranoid, rumors were spread in school that I was diseased and contagious. In my memory, kids would gasp and point when they saw my unsightly hands. Even a few teachers nervously kept their distance. I weakly replied to anyone who would listen that it was eczema, a genetic dry skin condition, and it was **not** contagious. My sense of deep shame of my skin's sensitivity deepened my larger sense of shame for who I was and my unkempt, seemingly poverty-stricken state. It took me years, decades even, to unravel the fact that my siblings and I had not, in reality, been poor; rather, we were children of extremely intelligent but poorly socialized parents, one a workaholic who put his ambition and career ahead of his family, and the other a stay-at-home mom who likely had undiagnosed, and thus untreated, high-functioning autism. Or rather, our poverty was indeed real, heartbreakingly so, but it was not so much of the financial sort so much as cultural and spiritual impoverishment.

My siblings and I had inherited our parents' traumas and their families' traumas; and they, as products of materialistic, rationalist, industrialized, individualist, and academic cultures, unconsciously manifested and projected their own traumas onto us. I had always struggled with feeling othered, not only from our impoverished, neglected upbringing, but also from my larger features and my wild, untameable hair. I thought of myself as white, but I also viscerally felt that I wasn't quite white enough; I knew I was always also "other." Many of my peers and teachers automatically assumed I was Jewish, which I tended to resent and deny. Though I largely rejected the label throughout my youth as my parents were secular, and we were brought up with little Jewish religious influence (despite having celebrated some Jewish holidays and growing up eating an array of Jewish cuisine throughout our upbringing), in adulthood I have come to recognize that Judaism is more than a religion, and it is an integral part of my identity. As first-generation American on my dad's side via Uruguay and Jewish-American on my mom's side, I have come to recognize that my identity exemplifies the complexity of identity politics; my background is 100% European/Caucasian, yet historically, my heritage was not considered white from either of my parental lineages, being primarily of Ashkenazi Jewish lineage on my mom's side and primarily of Italian ethnic lineage on my dad's side.

I couldn't help but to feel ashamed of my genes, with my sensitive skin and unruly hair from my dad's side and my large features that aren't conventionally white from both sides of my family. I had a persistent sense of otherness growing up, and there was nothing I so painfully wanted as to fit in.

The state of my skin aggravated and deepened my larger sense of shame, deep unworthiness, and otherness. It served to me as yet more proof that I was fundamentally inferior and unworthy, that I would never be good enough; my hair was too curly and unruly, my eyebrows too big, my parents were too poor and negligent, and my skin was defective. For years I harbored anger and resentment toward my dad, blaming him for passing on defective genes to me. It was *his* fault that I had to live with such an embarrassing — and painful — condition, I thought, and I resented this immensely. Yet I also recognized it wasn't anything he'd intentionally passed on to me, for though I would mope to him about my eczema and me feeling cursed for my skin's sensitivity, I never outright blamed him.

In high school, determined to put aside my preoccupation with my skin, I decided to pursue my interest in pottery. My senior year, I eagerly went to a pottery studio almost every day after classes, where I would lose myself in making large sculptures and pots. My hands suffered, but I was too busy and focused on my artistic creations to care. Even now, despite the perils to my skin that working with clay caused, I look back fondly and nostalgically on those days of intense artistic absorption. Likely, the soothing and centering activity of working with clay was enough to offset its drying effects on my skin; with my improved state of mental health arising from this hobby, my inflammation was minimized. The clay also likely contained minerals that helped my skin, even while it also dried it.

6

So when my friends in high school were battling with depression and anxiety and were trying different prescriptions, I barely thought to consider them. I felt unworthy and intrinsically and irrefutably inferior, doomed to a life of unworthiness and inferiority. I was resigned to feeling such a profound sense of unworthiness that I similarly felt resigned to a deep-seated feeling of grief beyond repair. Yet at the same time, I had always been interested in spirituality and religions. Raised by a Jewish mother mostly in a secular manner because of her disavowal of her mother (with whom she'd had a strained relationship due to her mother not being culturally equipped to address her daughter's mental illness), and because of my dad's very academic-driven identification as an atheist, my childhood left me wanting to find spirituality and meaning. I hungered for something more, and I sensed it was out there.

In high school, influenced by the 90's D.A.R.E. (Drug Abuse Resistance Education) culture and my parents' general abstention from alcohol and weed, I stayed away from substances, convinced they were deleterious. By college, however, I began experimenting. My first strong experience with weed, in the form of a brownie, brought me to a very altered state of consciousness where I simply shed my self-consciousness and was in short, very high. At one point, I was sitting with a circle of people gathered around me, enacting an imaginary caricatured conversation between a grandmother and grandfather. While some of my peers had found me hilarious (rightfully so, I believe), others thought perhaps I might be schizophrenic and that I should stay away from substances accordingly. Yet for me personally, the event had been cathartic; it was the first time, without alcohol, that I was able to live fully in myself, to lose a sense of my ego and self-consciousness, to engage with others without having a profound sense of my own self and my perceived sense of lacking and unworthiness.

I didn't try psychedelics until my senior year of college, during which time I'd had strong, profound experiences on both acid and mushrooms but found mushrooms to be my preferred substance. On acid I'd had my first and only real difficult trip: first, feeling overwhelmed and claustrophobic from the energy in a crowded room where music with a thumping bass line was blaring too loudly and insistently in my altered state, and then afterward, having fled to the quietude of the outdoors, feeling overwhelmed by the immensity of the night sky and all it revealed. Thankfully, I was able to refocus my energy productively and channel it into painting for the remainder of the acid trip, but those feelings of being overwhelmed by the intensity and duration of the trip have left me more cautious about LSD and drawn more to the natural experiences fostered by "magic" mushrooms, or psilocybin mushrooms.

It would be remiss of me to not mention that I did try SSRI's on multiple occasions—in college and then multiple times since. I never managed to adjust to them and also suffered from harsh side effects (sudden cystic acne and brittle, dry hair, among others). I am grateful for my body so vehemently rejecting these pharmaceuticals, as I had always been skeptical of them and their role in actually helping to "heal" and "treat" depression and anxiety. If two-thirds of the population were prone to depression and anxiety, I could recognize these states and the accompanying existential dread to be an intrinsic part of the human condition. Yet my solution at the time was to drink alcohol excessively, smoke pot socially, and to recklessly pursue intimate connections while inebriated.

While I had ongoing periods of relief from my eczema flare-ups, my skin continued to plague me through college and beyond, though thankfully during my college years it was mostly only my hands that suffered. I stopped being vegan my second year of undergraduate studies, and my hands seemed only slightly more prone to flare-ups. I had my tendency toward eczema under control, or so it seemed. For awhile. Unfortunately, true to typical college traditions, I began partying and taking care of myself less, which further aggravated my skin.

With the escalation of my drinking my first year out of college, I began getting dry patches I had never before experienced. On one occasion, I was sure that I had contracted ringworm. On the side of my stomach was a raised, reddish circle. Panicked, I went to the drugstore, where I showed a pharmacist; he looked at my skin dubiously and said it didn't appear to be ringworm. All the same, he found me an anti-fungal cream and advised me to see a doctor if the rash didn't improve or disappear in a few days. Sure enough, my skin soon became more inflamed. I promptly booked an appointment at the doctor's office; and the doctor quickly determined what my red circle was. "Hmm," he murmured. "Interesting. What you have there is nummular eczema. It simply means eczema that occurs in a circle. Usually, it occurs more in elderly populations." *Huh*. Was I taking care of myself that badly? He prescribed me a strong topical steroid, a more potent formula than the kind I'd been using for my usual eczema flare-ups. The "ringworm" patch soon faded and eventually went away entirely, though my skin remains slightly discolored there, having less pigmentation where the eczema once was. While the topical steroid worked in this case, I soon realized that I was becoming too dependent on using these medicated creams on my hands. My skin seemed to be thinning there; alarmed, I learned with further research that long-term use of topical steroids does indeed cause the skin to become weaker and thinner. Yet I continued to rely on this approach of moisturizers and topic steroid creams and gels for over a decade. I did not yet understand nor was I yet ready to shift toward a holistic approach toward self-care and self-healing.

Though I'd experienced a profound spiritual awakening the first time I had tried psilocybin "magic" mushrooms in college, and my first exposure to this sacrament was a magical, mystical experience, I had no knowledge of how to integrate what I had experienced and still struggled immensely with my own demons. I casually, recreationally came back to mushrooms a handful of times in my 20's but did not regularly use them as I did not have easy or reliable access to them. And NYC in the early 2000's was very much a culture that promoted drinking. I was here for it.

I allowed the power of the mushroom sacrament to largely fade from my view as it was likewise still suppressed in larger society. I allowed myself to be consumed by my lifestyle and the party culture of NYC. And though I longed to have that magic mushroom experience again and often fondly remembered the life-changing mystical experiences that the mushrooms had granted me access to, I had not fully been equipped to integrate the knowledge and wisdom I had gained from these experiences.

Not having easy access to psilocybin mushrooms further steered me toward my party-girl NYC ways that I very quickly became habituated to. I struggled with notions of worthiness left over from multi-layered childhood trauma, and surely from not only my individual traumas but also from intergenerational trauma as a Jewish-American on one side and as a first-generation American on the other, that I was also not entirely consciously re-enacting throughout most of my time of living in NYC as I stayed within my comfort zones. I allowed myself to get caught up in the hustle and bustle of NYC, knowing I was living without real purpose but also feeling helpless to change. I continued to seek out both fun and obliteration via alcohol and weed primarily, during college and up through my 20's and even early 30's. My life was one of escapism, living a reckless life to compensate for everything I'd felt lacking in my childhood and to fill my void of real purpose and meaning.

I had moved to NYC in August 2003 in my early 20's, and I had clocked over 15 years living there, entangled in the madness that is (or was) both living in NYC and early adulthood -- and early womanhood in the early 2000's, more specifically. The city, an addictive, fickle, tempestuous, and demanding lover, imprinted itself upon me, and gradually but also suddenly, I began finding myself being pulled like a pool floatie in erratic currents between shifting, overlapping, and contradictory facets of it as I continued to come up for air and then re-immerse myself in the city and all of its hyped-up madness. I dreaded the black outs and hangovers, but the alcohol-fueled partying gave me the release I craved. I had come to rely on the release of alcohol and mostly convinced myself that my drinking was not problematic, that I was not an alcoholic, as I drank only socially and was a happy, funny, charming drunk. It was what people did.

But time marched on, as it does, and as alcohol became harder on my system, I began veering away from it and started increasingly taking MDMA, mushrooms, and synthetic psychedelics. The shift away from alcohol, while healthy, was coupled with a shift toward harsher chemicals. The chemicals from the MDMA and the synthetic psychedelics, coupled with the inflammatory foods I was still consuming, propelled not only my eczema to flare up but for my skin to react viscerally, with acne and bacterial infections across my chest and face for weeks on end. My eczema suddenly began to flare up in new places, inching up my arms and clustering with angry, itchy patches around my ankles as never before. I decided to seek the help of an acupuncturist. Having never visited an acupuncturist before, I was slightly taken aback by the entire experience, and continued to feel slightly discomfited by it during my second two visits. While I am still on the fence about the actual pins and needles of acupuncture, I am grateful for the insights my acupuncturist offered. We went over my lifestyle, dietary and health habits. She advised me to use non-soap cleansers, which I try to do, and to eliminate wheat and/or dairy from my diet. I continue to consume both, but I do so much more sparingly than in the past. Though I have not cut out wheat, dairy, or meat entirely, I have drastically minimized how much I consume these types of foods as well as processed foods in general. I have learned to skew more toward a plant-based diet, one rich in nuts and seeds, to help minimize inflammation and help promote healthy skin and overall good health. I also decided that I would seriously moderate my drinking, roughly when I was 32 years old. And this decision is probably what has helped my skin the most.

My only explanation for why I didn't cut down on drinking sooner is that old habits are hard to break. My acupuncturist also prescribed me Chinese medicinal herbs, which I could never entirely stomach. "They taste a little gross, right?" she asked me. "We — Americans — aren't used to bitterness," she explained. That didn't make it any easier, though, to stomach the herbs. I snuck honey into my Chinese herbal tea, but I still haven't managed to finish it, years later.

Finally, my acupuncturist also suggested several supplements to take: Vitamin B-Complex (which can ease stress and therefore prevent the urge to itch), turmeric, flaxseed oil, and Vitamin E. Additionally, I decided to take Açaí supplements and probiotics. While I'm not always consistent with taking them, the supplements have seemed to help. Even if there's a placebo effect happening, at least it's happening.

With further research, I also learned of Elidel, a brand of topical immuno-modulator cream that suppresses the immune system where eczema flare-ups occur. As eczema is often a result of an overactive immune system, the cream works to calm down the flare-up by suppressing the immune response, and it is recommended for people whose skin does not respond to topical cortisone creams or who want an alternative without the harsh side effects of cortisone creams. I went to the doctor yet again for my skin, insisting that I be prescribed Elidel. "Unfortunately, it's under patent, so you'll have to pay $70 out of pocket." Yikes. But what could I do — I agreed. The new cream seemed to help me, though I also occasionally got secondary infections when I used it, as a lowered immune system makes your skin — especially dry, cracked skin — more susceptible to viruses and bacteria. So I no longer use Elidel regularly either. I still have topical cortisone and Elidel creams that I use in case of a severe flare-up, but I have focused on preventing and minimizing flare-up through eating well, staying hydrated, avoiding liquor and large quantities of dairy and wheat, minimizing stress, and keeping both moisturizer and anti-itch creams handy. In short, I've learned to take on a holistic, preventative approach.

Eczema is a condition that I will always have, but I have learned to minimize flare-ups and to become empowered to take a holistic, preventative approach. **I have learned as well that eczema itself is not the problem, even; it**

is a symptom of not living a healthy, balanced life. By living a healthier, more well-balanced, and happier life, by taking care of myself, I am able to mostly keep the eczema at bay. I have learned as well that cannabis and mushrooms (both psychoactive and non-psychoactive mushrooms) are tremendous tools in helping the body to heal and to maintain health and wellness.

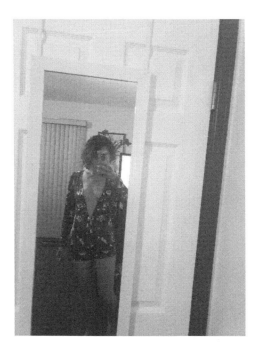

(Author, above, in fox and mushroom jumper; image courtesy of author)

The lines for me with substances have always been blurred between recreational and spiritual use. As I believe all dichotomies are, I have found that dichotomy to be false for me personally, as what was for me recreational and spiritual bled and spilled into each other. As I have evolved through time, I am so grateful to have gained knowledge of and access to cannabis and psilocybin mushrooms. I have found them key for my healing and wellness, key for me to not stay mired in grief from the traumas of my childhood, the traumas of living in a toxic, disconnected and patriarchal society, and the traumas of experiencing the deaths of multiple loved ones.

On some levels, I had always lived authentically to myself. I had never envisioned a 9-5 desk job for myself, though I did manage to hold a few down over the years, drawn by both the cultural and financial incentives. Still, I managed to manifest the artist life, balancing childcare work, teaching in various capacities, and selling art with working across the spectrum of sex work (SW), but in ways I believed would always keep me mostly anonymous: being a sugar baby, escort, erotic massage artist, and play party hostess. My personal and professional selves soon bled into each other as I gave into hedonism head-first, or perhaps more accurately put, with an open heart and an open pussy. With my sacral chakra. Yet I still relied heavily on alcohol for many of those years and did not fully give into my power or recognize my divine female power or strengths as I let my insecurities and childhood traumas fester.

Part of my living the unconventional life and my reckless pursuit with SW related to my sense of unworthiness and my childhood traumas. On one hand, SW allowed me to be empowered and take control of my sexuality. It allowed me to live a life less burdened by the 9-5 routine and have more free time, a commodity I valued more than money. SW also was instrumental to me in surviving on my own terms in my 20's and early 30's in this mechanized, patriarchal society. As a person with a sensitive immune system, with eczema and allergies exacerbated by stress, cold weather, my traumas, and hormonal fluctuations, SW allowed me to control my work schedule and rest according to my body's needs. I recognize here that my lighter complexion and longer-limbed physique were enormously advantageous to my adventures and exploits in SW. Yes, SW can be exploitative; all labor is. What was problematic about my SW was also that it was inhibiting me from living my more authentic, purpose-driven life; but that is also a challenge presented by the nature of capitalism. As such, I believe it is immensely important for SW to be decriminalized and destigmatized, for the safety and well-being of our collective society.

To be sure, I was reckless and put myself at risk numerous times. I am lucky I managed to leave SW behind and not have caught any untreatable, long-term STIs from the risky behavior I engaged in. I am profoundly lucky and privileged to never have had a run-in with law enforcement. I was not always great at setting boundaries, yet this is a quandary I feel that is faced universally in intimate connections with men. I definitely had a few encounters during my SW journey in which I was disrespected, but I never felt actively harmed. I was generally able to understand any man's disrespect as his own projections and issues. In all honesty, also, I had much more traumatizing experiences throughout my dating pursuits than from my SW pursuits. Which is not to mitigate the positive relationships and experiences I had either. Yet I believe my difficulties in making more meaningful, well-developed connections related to the superficial culture of NYC. My lifestyle in NYC granted me the freedom of having multiple selves while also making it impossible for me to practice radical honesty with myself and/or in my relationships. Of course, it took the pain of going through this way of living and the development of hindsight to recognize this.

I am so profoundly grateful that I was able to — quite literally — flee NYC during the first peak of the coronavirus pandemic in June 2020. Fast forward to the present, and I am now wealthier and wiser than when I began that addictive, volatile affair with NYC but with less social cache and freedom, and of course less of that youthful, innocent optimism than I had in that hazy because now-so-distant but yet also crystal-clear, rose-colored and alcohol-fueled youth of my 20's. Yet I also feel wiser, more empowered, more comfortable with myself — even if terrified of the future and what it may hold for myself, for my daughter, and for humanity and the larger natural world.

I can and do lament the mistakes and foolhardy passions and illusions of my youth; I mourn my directionlessness, my recklessness, and the time and energy wasted. I mourn that I let myself wallow in immaturity and a profound sense of lack of purpose. Yet I also feel grateful that I've come out alive, quite literally so as I mourn friends who have passed away from struggles with mental illness, alcohol, and substance use. I continue to live to honor the spirits of those who I've known and loved who are no longer with us in physical form, and I hold that much more perspective and wisdom because of all that I've witnessed, experienced, and endured. I am learning to understand and experience platitudes like "love is all there is," learning to practice mindfulness, gratitude, and being present with myself, with my daughter, and with the state of this world in all of its beauty and all of its pain.

Motherhood was one of the key stepping stones in helping me to break my ungrounded ways of living promoted by the NYC party and nightlife culture of the time, though I had begun pivoting away from my reckless relationship with alcohol shortly before pregnancy. As I matured into my 30's, it became apparent to me that drinking heavily was no longer serving me, and I learned to largely replace the urge to drink with my growing affinity for cannabis and psychedelics. But even learning to steer away from synthetic products and break unhealthy behavioral patterns was a process that took me time; I needed to hit the low points to learn to respect my body's needs.

It was only in my late 30's, through the new lens of motherhood, and thanks to greater economic freedom from a rent buy-out and then life insurance benefits from my father's passing, that I was able to really begin to approach my healthcare more holistically. Western medicine has indeed produced powerful tools to treat a variety of ailments and conditions, but it has fallen short in its myopic approach that treats symptoms rather than addressing causes. I have begun a functional mushroom regime together with a primarily plant- and fungi-based diet that has immensely, miraculously helped minimize my immune response. Not only has my skin drastically improved, but my immune system, my overall energy level, and my sense of self have transformed and experienced healing beyond what I had ever imagined to be possible.

Over the years I had a few run-ins with cannabis that left me in an awful state of feeling, quite literally, too high, puking from nausea, and having to pass out just from feeling too stoned. Yet I knew and trusted to always come back to the plant, as I recognized and continue to recognize that cannabis has immense therapeutic use. It has aided me in managing my anxiety and in connecting with the rhythms of myself and of music, through dancing, through humor, through explorations of mind and body. I am thankful now for the growing decriminalization of cannabis and the growing recognition of its medicinal values. Likewise, I am grateful to have access to amounts with clear dosages so I know not to take too much, and I have a general sense of what to expect from what I take.

Yet I have also witnessed the ways in which the stigmatization of cannabis has prevented those who may most need its help, those of the "I don't want to lose power of my mind or diminish my mental focus" persuasion and those of the "but I have an addictive personality" persuasion, who are still repulsed even by trying the non-psychotropic forms of the plant due to decades of incessant political "anti-drug" lobbying and policing and their reciprocal distrust accordingly of the plant and its medicinal properties. There is a middle ground, and the best way to help people develop a healthy relationship to cannabis is to decriminalize it and spread education around its therapeutic uses. As Ricki Lake made poignant in the documentary she co-produced, "Weed the People," which explored the potential of cannabis to help children battling cancer, the work was not really about cannabis at all but rather about helping people to become empowered to heal themselves. As I have learned in Merry Jane's *The CBD Solution*, medical students sadly are still largely not trained in the healing properties of cannabis. Yet its therapeutic potential has already been recognized for a vast number of auto-immune and inflammatory ailments that traditional pharmaceuticals have never been capable of treating well, from eczema and allergies to fibromyalgia to migraines. I believe that, with this growing green wave of cannabis's decriminalization and legalization, the plant's medical value will increasingly become apparent to the mainstream as well.

Though I find cannabis to be the most helpful substance for me to use in terms of frequency, psilocybin mushrooms are the substance that I find to be the most profound. Rekindling my relationship with psychedelics and more specifically, finding my home, myself, and my power again with the help of psilocybin and cannabis, has been truly revolutionary for me as I rebuild myself in this chapter of my life. Through my intentional use of cannabis and psychedelics, I have been able to release traumas and my associated negative mindset and behavioral patterns that no longer serve me. I have developed a healthier relationship with myself and my body, and I've become more conscious and intentional about how I care for my body and myself through the food and substances I consume. I have added regular functional mushroom usage to my regimen, enjoying both gourmet mushrooms and mushroom supplements (capsules and tinctures) on a regular basis, and doing so has had startling effects for me in the degree to which it has strengthened my immune system and minimized my inflammation and allergies.

I feel compelled to be an advocate for plant and mushroom substances in what I believe is the dawn of a re-emergent, earth-based, mycelial era. I full-heartedly believe that cannabis and fungi, among others, are natural substances from the earth that we as humans have co-evolved with. Likewise, I full-heartedly believe that the use of any natural substances is our natural-born right, and that the stigmatization of, criminalization of, lack of access to, and suppression of knowledge about these substances among the wider population generally, and more specifically among marginalized people, is a complete travesty and gaping injustice that we must work together to undo, as we collectively mourn in this time of pandemic and late-stage capitalism. Nature (plant and fungi medicines) and sex (sex work) urgently need to be destigmatized and decriminalized in this time of exacerbated mental health and economic struggles, for our individual and collective healing and well-being.

As I have been progressing through my healing journey, I've been so grateful to learn how profoundly cannabis and psilocybin mushrooms are sacraments for the body, the mind, and the soul; they are literally medicines that help promote neurogenesis and thereby help us to maintain wellness and be the best versions of ourselves. I am also learning and understanding more as time unfolds that paradox is at the heart of existence. I have always been worthy, even if I have always struggled to see myself as so. I have always been a goddess, even if I have also been a whore (and the goddess/whore dichotomy is a false one). I have always been able to heal myself, even as I have struggled to find and give light to my power. And as I am continuing to grow into my power and lean into my worthiness and my divine connections with this earth, myself, and with humanity and all of the earth's beings, I want to help others to realize their own potential for healing, in this time when we most need to develop our relationship to ourselves, to each other, and to the planet, for our individual and our collective healing. Our earth has the medicines we need, we just need to trust them and ourselves.

Stay connected:

Twitter @healinglivmama

IG: @healinglivmama (personal) and
@wellnessawakeningllc (professional)

FB: https://www.facebook.com/groups/wellnessawakeningllc

Linktree: https://linktr.ee/healinglivmama

REFERENCES AND FURTHER RESOURCES ON HOLISTIC HEALTH

Ashraf S. A. et al. (June 2020). "Cordycepin for Health and Wellbeing: a Potential Bioactive Bioactive Metabolite of an Entomopathogenic Medicinal Fungus *Cordyceps* with Its Nutraceutical and Therapeutic Potential." *Molecules.* https://www.ncbi.nlm.nih.gov/pmc/articles/PMC7356751/

Bourzat, Françoise. (2019). Consciousness Medicine: Indigenous Wisdom, Entheogens, and Expanded States of Consciousness for Healing and Growth. North Atlantic Books.

Canal, C. E., & Murnane, K. S. (2017). The serotonin 5-HT2C receptor and the non-addictive nature of classic hallucinogens. *Journal of Psychopharmacology (Oxford, England)*, *31*(1), 127–143. http://doi.org/10.1177/0269881116677104

Carhart-Harris, R. L. & Goodwin, G. M. (2017). The Therapeutic Potential of Psychedelic Drugs: Past, Present and Future. *Neuropsychopharmacology*, https://doi.org/10.1038/npp.2017.84.

Carhart-Harris, R.L, Roseman, L., Bolstridge, M., Demetriou, L., et al. (2017). "Psilocybin for treatment-resistant depression: fMRI-measured brain mechanisms." Scientific Reports. 1307. https://doi.org/10.1038/s41598-017-13282-7

Griffiths, R.R., Richards, W.A., Johnson, M..W., et al. (2008). "Mystical-type experiences occasioned by psilocybin mediate the attribution of personal meaning and spiritual significance 14 months later." Journal of Psychopharmacology.22: 6, 621–632. https://doi.org/10.1177/026988110809430

Griffiths, R.R., Johnson, M., Carducci, M. et al. (2016). "Psilocybin produces substantial and sustained decreases in depression and anxiety in patients with life-threatening cancer: A randomized double-blind trial." Journal of Psychopharmacology. 30: 12, 1181–1197. https://doi.org/10.1177/0269881116675513

Griffiths, R.R. (2017, May 10). "John Hopkins Psilocybin Research Project: Studies of mystical experience, adverse effects, meditation in healthy volunteers, and palliative effects in cancer patients — implications for spirituality and therapeutics." [Video file]. Retrieved from https://www.youtube.com/watch?list=PL4F0vNNTozFSw5gRe_zVTAvNIwjYD_AIU&v=6bu3q3GMHfE

Grob, C.S., Danforth, A.L., Chopra, G.S., Hagerty, M, McKay, C.R., Halberstadt, A.L. et al. (2009). "A pilot study of psilocybin treatment in advanced-stage cancer patients with anxiety." Arch Gen Psychiatry. 68(1): 71–78. https://doi.org/10.1001/archgenpsychiatry.2010.116

Hasler, F., Grimberg, U., Benz, M.A. et al. (2004). "Acute psychological and physiological effects of psilocybin in healthy humans: a double-blind, placebo-controlled dose-effect study.

28

Psychopharmacology. 172: 145. https://doi.org/10.1007/s00213-003-1640-6

Hendricks, P.S., Johnson, M.W., Griffiths, R.R. (2015). "Psilocybin, psychological distress, and suicidality." Journal of Psychopharmacology. 29: 9, 1041–1043. https://doi.org/10.1177/0269881115598338

Isokauppila, Tero. (March 14, 2019). The healing power of mushrooms [video]. YouTube. https://www.youtube.com/watch?v=VZnGwFblXpA&ab_channel=TalksatGoogle

Keremedchiev, Simeon. (Dec. 21, 2016). "Psychedelics: effects on the human brain and physiology." [video file]. TEDx Talks. Retrieved from https://www.youtube.com/watch?v=FyAgx_tzh80&t=37s&ab_channel=TEDxTalks

Lake, Ricki & Epstein, Abby. (2018). Weed The People [video]. https://www.weedthepeoplemovie.com/

Maroon, J., Bost, J. (April 26, 2018). "Review of the neurological benefits of phytocannabinoids." 9:91. Retrieved from: http://surgicalneurologyint.com/surgicalint-articles/review-of-the-neurological-benefits-of-phytocannabinoids/

Maté, Gabor, M.D. (January 19, 2021). "How Childhood Trauma Leads to Addiction." [video file]. Retrieved from https://www.youtube.com/watch?v=BVg2bfqblGI&ab_channel=AfterSkool

Maté, Gabor, M.d. (2010). In the Realms of Hungry Ghosts: Close Encounters with Addiction. North Atlantic Books.

Merry Jane. Wilson, Laura, Ed. The CBD Solution. Wellness: How Cannabis, CBD, and Other Plant Allies Can Change Your Everyday Life. Chronicle Books: San Francisco.

Pollan, M. (2018). How to Change Your Mind: What the New Science of Psychedelics Teaches Us About Consciousness, Dying, Addiction, Depression, and Transcendence. https://www. penguinrandomhouse.com/books/529343/how-to-change-your-mind-by-michael-pollan/

Powell, Martin. (2010). Mushrooms: The Essential Guide. Mycology Press.

Powell, Martin. (June 6, 2018). Why all mushrooms are magic [video]. YouTube. https://www. youtube.com/watch?v=fITifKJwZZc&ab_channel=BrightonNaturalHealthCentre

Shahzad, F., Anderson, D., & Najafzadeh, M. (2020). The antiviral, anti-inflammatory effects of natural medicinal herbs and mushrooms and SARS-CoV-2 Infection. *Nutrients*, *12*(9), 2573. https://doi.org/10.3390/nu12092573

Sheldrake, Merlin. (2020). Entangled Life: How Fungi Make Our Worlds, Change Our Minds & Shape Our Futures. Penguin Random House LLC.

Stamets, Paul. (January 13, 2021). "Psilocybin Mushroom Medicines: A Paradigm Shift in Global Consciousness." 2020 Bioneers Conference. Retrieved from https://www.youtube.com/watch?v=smBMn-CV9KF&ab_channel=Bioneers

Studerus, E., Krometer, M., Hasler, E. et al. (2010). "Acute, subacute and long-term subjective effects of psilocybin in healthy humans: a pooled analysis of experimental studies." Journal of Psychopharmacology. 25: 11, 1434–1452. https://doi. org/10.1177/0269881110382466

See also —

https://chacruna.net

http://www.maps.org/resources/papers

https://thethirdwave.co/

http://psychedelicscience.org/videos

Made in the USA
Coppell, TX
29 May 2021

56506955R10023